Contents

INTRODUCTION 4
LOW FIBER DIET 6
FOODS TO EAT 8
   Low-fiber foods 10
   Low-fiber end result 11
   Low-fiber greens 12
FOODS TO KEEP AWAY FROM 13
WHY IS A LOW-FIBER DIET USEFUL? 17
HOW TO BEGIN EATING FIBER AGAIN 19
KNOW YOUR FIBERS 20
MEAL PLAN 22
   Breakfast: 22
   Mid-morning snack: 22
   Lunch: 23
   Mid-afternoon snack: 23
   Dinner: 24
TIPS 24
RECOVERY 26
LOW FIBER DIET COOKBOOK 27
   BAKED EGGS WITH TOMATOES AND MOZZARELLA . 27
   BANANA PANCAKES 30

BUFFALO CAULIFLOWER BITES 32

BUTTERNUT SqUASH AND APPLE SOUP 34

CANTALOUPE AND MINT GRANITA 37

CAULIFLOWER HUMMUS 40

CAULIFLOWER RICE WITH SAUTÉED VEGETABLES ... 42

CRANBERRY-STUFFED CHICKEN BREASTS 45

EDAMAME HUMMUS 48

GREEK YOGURT FETTUCCINI ALFREDO 49

GREEK-STYLE GRILLED CHICKEN 51

GREEN RANCH DRESSING 53

LIME AND COCONUT CHICKEN 55

MANGO LASSI 57

MEATLESS BLACK BEAN CHILI 58

PORTOBELLO MUSHROOM BURGERS 60

QUINOA SALAD WITH FETA 63

RED CABBAGE SLAW 66

SALMON FILLET WITH YOGURT AVOCADO SAUCE ... 68

SLOPPY TURKEY JOE SLIDERS 70

SPAGHETTI SqUASH CASSEROLE WITH BROCCOLI AND CHICKEN 73

SPICED CHICKPEAS 77

SWEET POTATO HASH 79

TORTILLA ESPAÑOLA 82

CONCLUSION 84

INTRODUCTION

Fiber is a substance in plant-based ingredients that remains undigested because it passes through the small gut. A low-fiber food regimen includes foods which are without difficulty digested and absorbed.

Following a low-fiber weight-reduction plan (also known as a low residue weight-reduction plan) reduces the quantity of undigested food shifting via the small gut, which reduces stool length and frequency. This is mainly critical for human beings with inflammatory bowel disorder (IBD) who are experiencing a flare-up.

People preparing for a colonoscopy may additionally want to follow a low-fiber weight loss program, depending on their doctor's guidelines.

With cautious planning, it is nonetheless possible to get all of the crucial nutrients from a spread of low-fiber meals.

In this book, we take a look at what ingredients to consist of and people to keep away from whilst following a low-fiber food regimen.

LOW FIBER DIET

A low-fiber weight loss plan (additionally known as a restricted-fiber weight loss plan) limits the amount of excessive-fiber foods you devour each day. This facilitates deliver your digestive system a rest. A low-fiber eating regimen should:

- lessen the quantity of undigested food shifting through your intestines and bowels
- ease the amount of labor your digestive system isn't doing
- lessen the amount of stool you produce
- ease stomach pain, diarrhea, and other symptoms

Only eat a low-fiber diet in case your physician tells you to. This is often to treat signs and symptoms like diarrhea and cramping, before colonoscopies, after certain surgical procedures, or if you have a flare-up of one of the following gut problems:

- irritable bowel syndrome
- diverticulitis
- Crohn's sickness
- ulcerative colitis

This food plan is proscribing, nutritionally limiting, and not meant for weight loss. If you don't do it right, it can purpose greater unintentional side effects and signs and symptoms in the end. Read greater to learn how to do a low-fiber food plan right.

FOODS TO EAT

Proper nutrition is important for the first-class control of IBD and other situations that affect the bowel.

Some people best observe a low-fiber food regimen for brief periods, while others may also use it as a protracted-term approach. Even if just following the eating regimen for a for a short time, it's far nevertheless essential to attempt to devour an expansion of foods.

Typically, a low-fiber diet limits fiber consumption to around 10 to fifteen grams according to day for each males and females. A low-fiber food plan is made up of meals you shouldn't devour in large quantities or rely upon in your fitness. This includes white bread, ice cream, and protein. As lengthy as you keep on with a low-fiber food regimen for a quick amount of time — till your bowels heal, diarrhea resolves, otherwise you're healed from surgery — you'll be OK.

The following meals may be protected as a part of a low-fiber diet, relying on individual signs and symptoms and tolerance:

Low-fiber foods

- white bread
- white pasta
- white rice
- foods made with subtle white flour, like pancakes
- low-fiber warm and bloodless cereal
- eggs
- nicely-cooked canned or clean veggies in small amounts
- potatoes without the pores and skin
- fat like olive oil, mayonnaise, gravy, and butter
- dairy merchandise if you could tolerate them

- gentle protein assets like eggs, tofu, fowl, and fish
- creamy peanut butter

Low-fiber end result

- fruit juices without pulp
- canned fruit
- bananas
- cantaloupe
- honeydew melon
- watermelon
- nectarines
- papayas
- peaches
- plums

Low-fiber greens

- nicely-cooked or canned vegetables without seeds or skins
- carrots
- beets
- asparagus tips
- white potatoes with out pores and skin
- string beans
- lettuce if you may tolerate it
- tomato sauces
- acorn squash with out seeds
- pureed spinach
- strained vegetable juice

You might also devour cucumbers with out seeds or pores and skin, zucchini, and shredded lettuce uncooked.

Any meals which you understand is hard to your system to deal with have to also be averted. When you're going on a low-fiber weight-reduction plan, sure meals — like spicy meals — may additionally have an effect on your digestive machine more. Tea, espresso, and alcohol may additionally want to be prevented during this time.

FOODS TO KEEP AWAY FROM

Foods to avoid on a low-fiber diet:

- Breakfast cereals, together with muesli, bran flakes, puffed wheat, shredded wheat, porridge, granola, or cereals with delivered dried culmination.
- Whole-wheat bread, seeded loaves, and bread with brought fruit, nuts, or seeds.
- All vegetable skins, peels, and seeds, together with potato skins.
- Whole-wheat or brown pasta or grains, which include brown or wild rice, bulgar wheat, quinoa, and couscous.
- Cakes or pastries with nuts, end result, or seeds, such as fig rolls, flapjacks, and fruit scones.

- Fruits with seeds and peels nonetheless connected, together with raspberries, strawberries, blueberries, blackcurrants, passion fruit, kiwi, oranges, coconut, and fresh figs.
- All dried fruit, together with figs, prunes, dates, and raisins.
- Any raw, raw veggies.
- Pulses, which include lentils, baked beans, kidney beans, and chickpeas.
- Seeds, including pumpkin, sunflower, and flaxseeds.
- Nuts, consisting of walnuts, brazil nuts, almonds, cashews, and crunchy peanut butter.

- Tough or fatty meat.
- Fish with bones and the skin nonetheless on.
- Caffeinated drinks, consisting of espresso, black tea, and cola.
- Chunky soups.

Ask your health practitioner approximately those meals and any other foods you're questioning approximately before you start the weight-reduction plan. Also make a factor to hold your fluid consumption excessive. This will help you avoid constipation even as on this healthy dietweight-reduction plan.

Always communicate on your health practitioner about your particular wishes and the form of plan with a view to maximum gain your normal health earlier than you hit the grocery keep. Make sure to study labels and avoid any food that incorporates greater than 1 gram of fiber.

You also can meet with a dietitian for particular meal plans and steering on ingesting a low-fiber food plan.

WHY IS A LOW-FIBER DIET USEFUL?

You must only pass on a low-fiber weight-reduction plan in case your physician tells you to. Your doctor might also advocate this food plan when you have:

- inflammatory bowel disease

- Crohn's disorder
- ulcerative colitis
- diverticulitis
- diarrhea
- stomach cramps
- constipation
- problem with digestion
- irritation or harm in your digestive tract
- narrowing of the bowel caused by a tumor
- put up-surgical recovery from gastrointestinal tactics like colostomy and ileostomy
- long gone via radiation or other kinds of treatments which would possibly have an effect on your gastrointestinal tract

You may additionally need to eat a low-fiber food regimen for 2 to three days prior to getting a colonoscopy.

HOW TO BEGIN EATING FIBER AGAIN

Once you've reset your digestive machine, you ought to slowly return to eating fiber-wealthy foods by means of introducing a small portion of one fiber food consistent with day. If the food doesn't purpose symptoms within 24 hours, it could be introduced in your weight loss program.

How much fiber you need is based to your age and intercourse.

	Adults (50 years or younger)	Adults (over 50)
men	38 g	30 g
ladies	25 g	21 g

Avoid ingesting all of your fiber in one sitting or meal. The satisfactory manner to get plenty of it's miles by means of consuming fruits with skins left on, raw vegetables, entire grains, beans, nuts, and seeds.

KNOW YOUR FIBERS

There are styles of fiber:

Soluble fiber meals soak up water during digestion, which turns them right into a gentle, gel-like substance. Soluble fiber meals, like apples, peas, or beans, are less annoying to the digestive tract and can regularly be eaten in small quantities.

Insoluble fiber ingredients don't dissolve completely within the stomach. The small bits of undigested meals that remain can be anxious to the intestines. On a low-fiber food regimen, you'll have to be specifically cautious to avoid foods like whole wheat, grains, and uncooked vegetables.

MEAL PLAN

Meal alternatives for someone following the low-fiber food regimen include:

Breakfast:

low-fiber cereal (for example Rice Krispies, Cornflakes, Special K) with milk or non-dairy milk

white bread or toast with butter and jelly

poached eggs

Mid-morning snack:

crumpet

clean yogurt or kefir

applesauce with cinnamon

Lunch:

a sandwich made from white bread with slices of turkey breast

white pasta with tuna

Mid-afternoon snack:

ripe banana

simple biscuits

pudding

canned mandarin oranges

Dinner:

white rice with salmon and coffee-fiber veggies

omelet

bird breast with mashed potato

TIPS

When introducing new foods, add only one at a time. This will assist a person perceive meals that make their signs worse.

Read the labels on pre-prepared or packaged food, as they'll include substances that cause signs and symptoms.

Avoid some thing with bits in it, such as yogurts, marmalade, mustard, popcorn, and crunchy peanut butter.

Here are a few more useful tips for an extremely low-fiber weight loss program:

- sieve soups and lumpy stews
- eat small meals each 3–four hours
- bite meals slowly and carefully
- keep away from huge quantities of caffeine or alcohol
- avoid wealthy sauces and spicy ingredients
- devour simplest small amounts of dairy
- avoid fizzy beverages

- communicate to a dietitian about what culmination and vegetables are secure to eat

RECOVERY

If eating or digestion remains difficult or painful, it is crucial to talk to a physician. People with IBD may additionally need significant guide from a dietitian to manipulate the ailment for the duration of times of relapse and remission.

While much studies is conflicting on the excellent nutritional method to save you or postpone IBD relapse, there may be a few proof that supports a semi-vegetarian weight-reduction plan and exclusion diets.

It is essential to eat a varied eating regimen that incorporates all the crucial nutrients and enough energy to preserve strength tiers.

LOW FIBER DIET COOKBOOK

BAKED EGGS WITH TOMATOES AND MOZZARELLA

Ingredients

- 2 tablespoons olive oil
- ½ small yellow onion, chopped
- 2 cloves garlic, minced

- 28-ounce can crushed tomatoes
- Salt and pepper
- 4 ounces fresh mozzarella, cut into 1/2-inch pieces
- ¼ cup fresh oregano leaves, coarsely chopped
- 8 eggs
- 4 slices multigrain toast (optional)

Instructions

- Thoroughly rinse fresh produce under warm running water for 20 seconds. Scrub to remove excess dirt.
- Preheat oven to 350 degrees.

- In a saucepan over medium-high heat, warm olive oil. Add onion and cook until translucent, about 5 minutes. Add garlic and cook until fragrant. Stir in tomatoes with juices, season with salt and pepper to taste, and bring to a boil. Reduce heat to low and simmer until nicely thickened, about 15 minutes. Season with more salt and pepper to taste.
- Place four medium ramekins on a baking sheet. Divide tomato sauce evenly between ramekins. Top with mozzarella and oregano. Break 2 eggs into each ramekin, on top of the tomato sauce and cheese, and season with salt and pepper.

- Bake until egg whites are opaque and yolks register as 160 degrees or higher using an instant-read thermometer (set but still slightly runny in the middle), about 15 minutes. Eggs will continue cooking from residual heat. Let cool slightly and serve with toast, if desired.

BANANA PANCAKES

Ingredients

- 2 large egg whites or ¼ cup liquid egg whites
- 1 ripe medium banana, mashed
- 2 tablespoons instant oats

- ¼ teaspoon cinnamon (optional)
- Cooking spray
- Sugar-free maple syrup, plain yogurt, or creamy nut butter (optional)

Instructions

- In medium bowl, whisk egg whites until frothy. Add banana, oats, and cinnamon, if using, and stir until combined.
- Heat large nonstick skillet over medium heat. Lightly coat pan with cooking spray. Spoon batter onto hot skillet to form three small pancakes. Cook until golden brown, about 2 to 3 minutes per side.
- Add any desired toppings.

BUFFALO CAULIFLOWER BITES

Ingredients

- Cooking spray
- 2 medium heads cauliflower, cut into small florets
- 1 cup brown rice flour, chickpea flour, or any flour available
- 1 cup water
- 2 teaspoons garlic powder
- 1 teaspoon salt
- 2 teaspoons butter
- 1 ⅓ cups Frank's Hot Sauce

Instructions

- Thoroughly rinse fresh produce under warm running water for 20 seconds. Scrub to remove excess dirt.

- Preheat oven to 450 degrees. Line a rimmed baking sheet with parchment paper or spray with cooking spray.

- Toss the cauliflower florets with flour, water, garlic powder, and salt. Place on prepared baking sheet and bake 20 minutes.

- In a small saucepan, melt butter with hot sauce. Pour butter mixture over baked cauliflower and toss to coat.

- Return cauliflower to oven and bake another 20 minutes. Internal temperature of cauliflower should be 145 degrees using an instant-read thermometer. Serve warm.

BUTTERNUT SqUASH AND APPLE SOUP

Ingredients

- 2½ cups butternut squash, peeled and cubed
- 4 tablespoons extra-virgin olive oil
- 1 yellow onion, chopped
- 1 clove garlic, minced
- 5 cups low-sodium vegetable stock
- 2 cups water
- 1 16-ounce can pumpkin puree

- 2 medium red apples, peeled and chopped
- ¼ teaspoon ground cinnamon
- ¼ teaspoon ground nutmeg
- ¼ teaspoon ground cloves
- ¼ teaspoon salt
- ½ teaspoon black pepper
- 4 tablespoons low-fat plain Greek yogurt
- Roasted pumpkin seeds (optional)

Instructions

- Thoroughly rinse fresh produce under warm running water for 20 seconds. Scrub to remove excess dirt.
- Preheat oven to 350 degrees.

- Line a rimmed baking sheet with parchment paper, then spread squash evenly on paper. Drizzle squash with 2 tablespoons olive oil and roast 8 to 10 minutes. Remove from oven and set aside.
- Heat remaining 2 tablespoons olive oil in a large pot over medium heat. Add onion and garlic. Cook until onion is soft and starts to brown. Add roasted squash, vegetable stock, water, pumpkin puree, apples, cinnamon, nutmeg, cloves, salt, and black pepper. Bring to a boil over high heat, then reduce to a simmer and cook until squash and apples are tender, about

20 minutes. Remove from heat and let cool.

- Puree soup using an immersion blender, food mill, food processor, or blender. Place pot over low heat until soup is warmed through, about 30 minutes. Add yogurt, stirring until completely combined. Soup should be 145 degrees using an instant-read thermometer.
- Ladle soup into bowls and garnish with seeds, if using.

CANTALOUPE AND MINT GRANITA

Ingredients

- 2 cups water
- 1 cup sugar, or more to taste
- 1¼ cup fresh mint leaves
- 1 cantaloupe, peeled, seeded, and chopped
- 3 tablespoons lime juice

Instructions

- Thoroughly rinse fresh produce under warm running water for 20 seconds. Scrub to remove excess dirt.
- In a small saucepan, combine the water, 1 cup sugar, and 1 cup mint leaves. Bring to a boil over medium heat. Reduce heat and simmer, stirring occasionally, until sugar has dissolved, about 5 minutes. Remove

pan from heat and set aside to cool, about 20 minutes. Pour cooled syrup through a strainer to remove mint leaves.

- In a blender, puree the strained syrup, cantaloupe, and lime juice until smooth, then taste. To sweeten more, add 1 tablespoon sugar at a time and blend; taste and repeat until desired flavor is reached. Add remaining mint leaves and blend until finely chopped.
- Pour the mixture into a 9x13 glass baking dish and freeze, at least 8 hours or overnight.

- Using the tines of a fork, scrape the granita to the desired texture and serve in chilled bowls.

CAULIFLOWER HUMMUS

Ingredients

- 1 medium head cauliflower, cut into small florets
- Cooking spray or oil
- 1 clove garlic
- ⅓ cup tahini (or cashew butter or sesame oil)
- 2 tablespoons olive oil, plus more for garnish

- Salt and pepper to taste
- 2 tablespoons parsley, for garnish
- 1 lemon, cut into wedges, for garnish

Instructions

- Preheat oven to 400 degrees. Line a rimmed baking sheet with parchment paper or spray with cooking spray.
- Place cauliflower florets on baking sheet. Coat with additional oil or cooking spray. Roast for 40 minutes, stirring halfway through. Remove from oven and let cool.
- In a food processor, combine cauliflower with garlic, tahini, lemon juice, olive oil, salt, and pepper. Process until smooth.

- Add water one tablespoon at a time for a thinner consistency, if desired.
- Transfer hummus to a bowl. Drizzle with olive oil and sprinkle with parsley, if desired.
- Serve with lemon wedges.

CAULIFLOWER RICE WITH SAUTÉED VEGETABLES

Ingredients

- 5 cups cauliflower florets (about 1½ heads cauliflower)
- 1 tablespoon olive oil
- 1 teaspoon minced garlic

- ½ red bell pepper, coarsely chopped into 1-inch pieces
- ½ yellow bell pepper, coarsely chopped into 1-inch pieces
- ½ zucchini, coarsely chopped into 1-inch pieces
- ½ yellow summer squash, coarsely chopped into 1-inch pieces
- Salt and pepper
- 2 tablespoons chicken broth

Instructions

- Thoroughly rinse fresh produce under warm running water for 20 seconds. Scrub to remove excess dirt, then set aside.

- Place cauliflower in a food processor and pulse several times until cauliflower resembles rice.
- Heat olive oil in a large skillet over medium-high heat. Add garlic and stir until fragrant, about 1 minute. Add bell peppers, zucchini, and squash. Season with salt and pepper to taste. Cook until vegetables begin to soften, stirring occasionally, about 5 to 7 minutes. Add cauliflower rice and chicken broth and stir well, until chicken stick reduces by half and vegetables are fully cooked. Internal temperature of cauliflower rice should be

145 degrees using an instant-read thermometer.

CRANBERRY-STUFFED CHICKEN BREASTS

Ingredients

- 1½ tablespoons plus 1 teaspoon olive oil
- 1 small apple, peeled and diced
- ½ cup dried cranberries
- 1 shallot, peeled and diced
- ¾ cup low-sodium chicken stock
- 4 boneless, skinless chicken breasts, about 4 to 6 ounces each
- ¼ cup balsamic vinegar
- Salt and pepper

Instructions

- Heat 1 teaspoon olive oil in a skillet over medium-high heat. Add apple and cook until tender, 3 to 4 minutes.
- In a small bowl, combine cooked apple, cranberries, shallot, and 1 tablespoon chicken stock. Set aside.
- Cut a deep horizontal pocket in the side of each chicken breast. Make the pocket as large as you can without piercing the top or bottom of the breast. Divide apple mixture evenly among chicken breasts, stuffing into each pocket. Secure pockets with toothpicks, threading along the side to close.

- Heat remaining 1½ tablespoons olive oil in a heavy skillet. Cook chicken, turning once, until golden brown. Add vinegar and remaining chicken stock, then bring to a boil. Lower heat and gently simmer chicken, turning once, 2 or 3 minutes per side.
- When chicken registers 165 degrees Fahrenheit or higher using an instant-read thermometer placed in the thickest part of the breast, remove from skillet and keep warm.
- Continue cooking sauce until reduced to a thick syrup. Season with salt and pepper to taste.

- Spoon sauce over chicken to serve.

EDAMAME HUMMUS

Ingredients

- 2 cups frozen shelled edamame
- 2 tablespoons tahini
- 2 cloves garlic, peeled
- 2 tablespoons olive oil
- 1 tablespoon cilantro leaves
- Juice of 2 lemons
- Salt and pepper

Instructions

- Thoroughly rinse fresh produce under warm running water for 20 seconds.

- Boil water in a medium saucepan. Add edamame and cook 1 to 2 minutes. Drain edamame and rinse under cold water to prevent it from cooking further.
- Add cooked edamame, tahini, garlic, olive oil, cilantro, and lemon juice to a food processor or blender and pulse until smooth. Add salt and pepper to taste.
- Serve immediately or transfer to an airtight container. Hummus can be stored up to 3 days in the refrigerator.

GREEK YOGURT FETTUCCINI ALFREDO

Ingredients

- 1 pound fettuccini
- 1½ cups whole-milk Greek yogurt
- ½ cup freshly grated Parmesan, plus more for serving
- 3 tablespoons minced garlic
- ¼ cup chopped fresh parsley
- 1 teaspoon pepper

Instructions

- Boil pasta in salted water per package instructions. Reserve 1 cup cooking liquid, then drain.
- Whisk together yogurt, ½ cup Parmesan, garlic, and parsley. Slowly whisk in cooking liquid a little bit at a time. Add

pepper. Pour sauce over pasta and toss to combine.

- Top with more Parmesan to taste and serve immediately. Pasta should register 145 degrees Fahrenheit or higher using an instant-thermometer placed in the middle of the dish.

GREEK-STYLE GRILLED CHICKEN

Ingredients

- ⅛ cup olive oil
- 3 cloves garlic, chopped
- 1 tablespoon fresh rosemary, chopped
- 1 tablespoon fresh thyme, chopped

- 1 tablespoon fresh oregano, chopped
- 2 lemons, juiced
- 4 boneless, skinless 5-ounce chicken breasts
- Oil for grill grate

Instructions

- In a large glass dish, mix olive oil, garlic, rosemary, thyme, oregano, and lemon juice. Add the chicken, spooning the mixture over it. Cover the dish, and marinate in the refrigerator 8 hours or overnight.
- Preheat grill on high heat.
- Lightly oil the grill grate. Place chicken on the grill, and discard marinade.

- Cook chicken pieces up to 6 minutes per side, until juices run clear and chicken is 165 degrees as measured by a meat thermometer.

GREEN RANCH DRESSING

Ingredients

- ½ cup light mayonnaise
- ½ cup plain Greek yogurt
- ½ tablespoon chopped fresh chives
- 1 teaspoon fresh parsley
- ¼ cup unsweetened almond milk
- 1 teaspoon lemon juice
- ½ teaspoon garlic powder

- ½ teaspoon onion powder
- 1 teaspoon fresh dill or ¼ teaspoon dried dill (optional)
- ¼ teaspoon sea salt
- ¼ teaspoon black pepper

Instructions

- Thoroughly rinse fresh produce under warm running water for 20 seconds.
- Add all ingredients to a blender. Blend until completely smooth. Add more almond milk, 1 tablespoon at a time, for a thinner consistency.
- Serve immediately or transfer to an airtight container. Dressing can be stored up to 3 days in the refrigerator.

LIME AND COCONUT CHICKEN

Ingredients

- 2 pounds boneless, skinless chicken breasts
- 1 lime
- 3 tablespoons vegetable oil
- ½ cup coconut milk
- 2 tablespoons low-sodium soy sauce
- 2 tablespoons sugar
- 2 teaspoons curry powder
- 1½ teaspoons ground coriander
- 1 teaspoon ground cumin
- 1½ teaspoons salt

- 4 tablespoons chopped fresh cilantro

Instructions

- Using a meat tenderizer, pound chicken breasts between sheets of wax paper until ⅛-inch thick.
- Zest lime into a large bowl; slice lime into wedges and set aside.
- Add oil, coconut milk, soy sauce, sugar, curry, coriander, cumin, and salt to zest and whisk to combine. Add chicken and toss to combine. Cover and refrigerate for 1 to 2 hours.
- Remove chicken, reserving marinade. Using a hot sauté pan, grill pan, or cast-iron skillet, brown chicken on both sides.

Chicken should register 165 degrees Fahrenheit using an instant-read thermometer inserted in the thickest part of the breast.

- Meanwhile, pour reserved marinade into a saucepan and bring to a boil. Reduce heat and simmer for 2 minutes, stirring to prevent burning.
- Serve sauce over chicken with cilantro and reserved lime wedges.

MANGO LASSI

Ingredients

- 2 cups chopped mango

- ½ cup whole-milk yogurt
- ½ cup coconut milk or whole milk
- 1 teaspoon lime juice
- 1 teaspoon honey
- Pinch of cardamom
- 6 ice cubes

Instructions

- Combine all ingredients in a blender. Pulse until smooth.

MEATLESS BLACK BEAN CHILI

Ingredients

- 1 medium onion, chopped
- 2 cloves garlic, minced or pressed

- 1 15-ounce BPA-free can low-sodium black beans, drained and rinsed
- 1 15-ounce BPA-free can no-salt-added diced tomatoes
- 1 tablespoon chili powder
- 1 tablespoon cumin
- 1 teaspoon unsweetened cocoa powder

Instructions

- Combine chopped onion and minced garlic in a bowl. Let sit for at least 5 minutes.
- Place all ingredients in a large pot and stir to combine. Cover and let simmer on low heat for about 20 minutes.
- Spoon into bowl and enjoy!

PORTOBELLO MUSHROOM BURGERS

Ingredients

- Cooking spray
- 3 tablespoons olive oil
- 1 small onion, finely chopped
- 6 cloves garlic, minced
- 1½ pounds portobello mushrooms, chopped
- 1 teaspoon red pepper flakes
- Salt and pepper
- 2½ cup bread crumbs (gluten free if desired)
- ½ cup grated carrots

- ⅓ cup green lentils, cooked
- 2 teaspoons dried parsley (optional)
- 2 teaspoons dried oregano (optional)
- 2 eggs, beaten

Instructions

- Thoroughly rinse fresh produce under warm running water for 20 seconds. Scrub to remove excess dirt.
- Preheat oven to 350 degrees. Coat a baking sheet with cooking spray.
- Heat a large skillet over medium-low heat. Add 1 tablespoon olive oil and onion. Sauté onion until soft. Add garlic, mushrooms, and red pepper flakes. Season with salt and pepper to taste.

Cook until mushrooms are brown, 5 to 8 minutes. Remove skillet from heat and transfer mushroom mixture to a large bowl to cool, at least 10 minutes.

- Add panko, breadcrumbs, carrots, lentils, and herbs to mushroom mixture. Season to taste with salt and pepper. Add eggs and stir to combine. Divide mixture into 8 patties.

- Reheat skillet over medium-low heat. Add the remaining 2 tablespoons olive oil. Cook each patty until golden brown, 3 to 4 minutes per side.

- Transfer patties to prepared baking sheet. Bake until cooked through, about 10 minutes. Internal temperature of patties should be 145 degrees using an instant-read thermometer. Serve warm.

QUINOA SALAD WITH FETA

Ingredients

- 2 cups quinoa
- 3½ cups low-sodium chicken or vegetable broth
- 1 cup grape tomatoes, halved
- ⅔ cup chopped fresh parsley
- ½ cup diced cucumber, peeled and seeded
- ½ cup minced red onions
- 4 ounces feta cheese, crumbled

- 3 tablespoons olive oil
- 3 tablespoons red wine vinegar
- 2 cloves garlic, minced
- Juice of 1 lemon
- Salt and pepper

Instructions

- Thoroughly rinse fresh produce under warm running water for 20 seconds. Scrub to remove excess dirt.
- Rinse quinoa in a fine-mesh colander under running water for at least 30 seconds. Drain well.
- In a saucepan, bring rinsed quinoa and broth to a boil. Reduce heat to medium-low, cover, and simmer until quinoa is

tender and broth is absorbed, 15 to 20 minutes. Transfer to a large bowl and set aside to cool.

- Add tomatoes, parsley, cucumber, onions, feta, olive oil, vinegar, and garlic to cooled quinoa and mix to combine. Pour lemon juice over quinoa salad and season with salt and pepper to taste. Toss to coat and refrigerate until ready to serve.
- Washing the quinoa well before cooking helps to remove bitterness caused by naturally occurring saponins. Saponins are chemical compounds found in quinoa and other plant-based foods, and have been

shown to possess a number of health benefits.

RED CABBAGE SLAW

Ingredients

- Cooking spray
- ½ cup pepitas or pumpkin seeds
- ½ cup sunflower seeds
- ½ head red cabbage, sliced thinly
- ½ jicama, peeled and chopped
- 1 mango (firm), sliced
- ¼ to ½ cup cilantro, chopped
- ½ cup pepitas or pumpkin seeds, toasted
- ½ cup sunflower seeds, toasted

- Juice from 2 limes

- ¼ cup rice wine vinegar

- 2 tablespoons honey

- ¼ cup extra-virgin olive oil

- Salt

Instructions

- Thoroughly rinse fresh produce under warm running water for 20 seconds. Scrub to remove excess dirt.

- Coat a skillet with cooking spray and toast seeds until brown, about 10 minutes.

- Combine toasted seeds, cabbage, jicama, mango, cilantro, lime juice, vinegar, honey, and olive oil in a large bowl. Add salt to taste.

- Serve immediately or transfer to an airtight container. Slaw can be stored up to 3 days in the refrigerator.

SALMON FILLET WITH YOGURT AVOCADO SAUCE

Ingredients

- 1 avocado
- ½ cup Greek yogurt
- 3 tablespoons cilantro leaves
- 1 clove garlic
- 2 tablespoons lemon juice
- 1 tablespoon water, plus more as needed
- 1 teaspoon salt, plus more for seasoning

- 1 teaspoon ground pepper, plus more for seasoning
- 4 3-ounce salmon fillets
- 1 tablespoons olive oil

Instructions

- Preheat oven to 400 degrees. Line a baking sheet with aluminum foil.
- Combine avocado, yogurt, cilantro, garlic, lemon juice, 1 tablespoon water, and 1 teaspoon each salt and pepper in a food processor and blend until smooth. If necessary, add more water, 1 tablespoon at a time, until sauce reaches desired consistency.

- Place fish skin-side down on prepared baking sheet. Season with salt and pepper and brush with olive oil. Bake fish until just cooked through, 8 to 10 minutes. Fish should register 145 degrees Fahrenheit using an instant-read thermometer in the middle of the fillet.
- Serve fish topped with sauce.

SLOPPY TURKEY JOE SLIDERS

Ingredients

- ½ cup carrot, minced
- 1 medium onion, diced
- ½ cup celery, minced

- 3 cloves garlic, minced
- 1 pound ground turkey
- 8-ounce can unsalted tomato sauce
- ½ cup ketchup
- 1 tablespoon brown sugar
- 1 teaspoon ground mustard
- 1 tablespoon Worcestershire sauce
- 1 tablespoon apple cider vinegar
- 1 teaspoon dried oregano
- ¼ teaspoon salt
- ⅛ teaspoon black pepper
- 5 whole-wheat hamburger buns

Instructions

- Thoroughly rinse fresh produce under warm running water for 20 seconds. Scrub to remove excess dirt.

- In a large saucepan or Dutch oven over medium-high heat, cook carrot, onion, celery, and garlic until onions are translucent. Add turkey, breaking it up with a wooden spoon, and cook until mostly browned. Drain excess liquid and fat. Set aside turkey mixture in pan.

- In a small bowl, whisk tomato sauce, ketchup, brown sugar, ground mustard, Worcestershire sauce, apple cider vinegar, oregano, salt, and pepper to combine. Pour sauce into pan with drained turkey mixture and stir until evenly coated. Cover and simmer 20 minutes, stirring occasionally. Sloppy joe mixture should register 165 degrees Fahrenheit or higher using an instant-read thermometer placed in the middle of the dish.

- Serve sloppy joe mixture in buns.

SPAGHETTI SQUASH CASSEROLE WITH BROCCOLI AND CHICKEN

Ingredients

- 4 pounds spaghetti squash, halved lengthwise and seeded
- 2 tablespoons water

- 1 tablespoon extra-virgin olive oil
- 4 cloves garlic, minced
- 1 pound chicken breast, diced
- 2 cups broccoli florets, chopped
- ½ cup low-sodium chicken broth
- 1½ cups grated part-skim mozzarella cheese
- ½ cup grated Parmesan
- 1 teaspoon Italian seasoning
- 1 teaspoon salt
- ¼ teaspoon ground pepper
- ¼ cup panko bread crumbs

Instructions

- Thoroughly rinse fresh produce under warm running water for 20 seconds. Scrub to remove excess dirt.
- Position racks in upper and lower thirds of oven; preheat to 375 degrees.
- Place squash cut-side down on a microwave-safe dish; add water and microwave on high until flesh is tender, 12 to 14 minutes. When cool, scrape flesh from rind in spaghetti like strands.
- Heat olive oil in a skillet over medium-high heat. Add garlic and chicken; cook until chicken is browned on all sides. Add broccoli and broth, and cook for 2 minutes.

- In a large bowl, toss shredded spaghetti squash and chicken mixture with ¾ cup mozzarella, 2 tablespoons Parmesan, Italian seasoning, salt, and pepper. Spread in an oven-safe casserole dish. Sprinkle with remaining ¾ cup mozzarella and 6 tablespoons Parmesan; top with bread crumbs.
- Bake on lower rack for 15 minutes. Move to upper rack and increase heat to 425 degrees. Bake until cheese browns, an additional 3 to 5 minutes. Casserole should register 165 degrees Fahrenheit or higher using an instant-read thermometer placed in the middle of the dish.

SPICED CHICKPEAS

Ingredients

- 1 teaspoon ground cumin
- 1 teaspoon smoked sweet paprika
- ½ teaspoon garlic powder
- ½ teaspoon onion powder
- ⅛ teaspoon salt
- ⅛ teaspoon black pepper
- Pinch of cayenne pepper
- 2 tablespoons extra-virgin olive oil
- 1 15-ounce can chickpeas, no salt added or low sodium, drained

Instructions

- Preheat oven to 400 degrees.

- In a medium mixing bowl, use a small whisk to combine cumin, paprika, garlic powder, onion powder, salt, black pepper, and cayenne. Add oil and whisk to combine.

- Place a double layer of paper towels on a work surface. Rinse chickpeas in a colander. Shake well, then spread chickpeas evenly across paper towels. Blot chickpeas using a clean paper towel. Repeat as needed, until chickpeas are thoroughly dry.

- Add chickpeas to spice mixture and, using your fingers, gently mix and massage until they are evenly coated.

- Line a baking sheet with parchment paper and spread chickpeas evenly across pan.

- Bake, rotating sheet every 8 minutes, until chickpeas are firm, 24 to 32 minutes.

- Remove sheet from oven and allow chickpeas to cool. Serve immediately or transfer to an airtight container. Chickpeas can be stored up to 3 days in the refrigerator.

SWEET POTATO HASH

Ingredients

- 2 tablespoons olive oil
- 4 sweet potatoes, peeled and shredded
- 1 bunch kale, chopped
- Salt and pepper
- Cooking spray
- 6 eggs

Instructions

- Thoroughly rinse fresh produce under warm running water for 20 seconds. Scrub to remove excess dirt.
- Preheat oven to 350 degrees.
- Heat a large skillet over high heat. Add olive oil and shredded sweet potato and cook until soft, about 10 minutes. Add

kale and cook until wilted. Season mixture with salt and pepper to taste.

- Coat a 9x13 baking dish with cooking spray. Spoon sweet potato mixture into prepared dish. Then, using a spoon, make 6 wells in the mixture, spaced evenly around the dish, and crack an egg into each one. Top with a sprinkle of salt and pepper.
- Bake until eggs are cooked and yolks are set. Internal temperature of the hash should be 160 degrees using an instant-read thermometer. Serve immediately.

TORTILLA ESPAÑOLA

Ingredients

- ¼ cup extra-virgin olive oil
- 2 Yukon Gold potatoes, peeled and grated
- 1 medium yellow onion, thinly sliced
- Salt and pepper
- 8 eggs

Instructions

- Preheat oven to 350 degrees.
- In a 10-inch cast-iron skillet or other large oven-safe skillet, heat 2 tablespoons olive oil over medium heat. Add potatoes and onion. Season with salt. Cook, stirring

occasionally, until onions are translucent. Set aside to cool; reserve skillet.

- When potato mixture is cool, whisk eggs in a large bowl, then add potato mixture and stir to combine. Season with salt and pepper.
- Wipe skillet, add remaining 2 tablespoons olive oil, and return to medium heat. Add egg mixture. Cook, gently shaking skillet as egg begins to set. With a rubber spatula, scrape along the sides of the skillet to prevent sticking.
- Once the sides are set, transfer skillet to oven. Bake about 15 minutes, making sure egg is cooked and not runny. Internal

temperature of tortilla española should be 160 degrees using an instant-read thermometer.

- Allow tortilla to sit in skillet for 10 minutes before serving. Serve in wedges.

CONCLUSION

Only devour a low-fiber food plan if your physician has advocated it. Your health practitioner might be able to inform you the way long you need to be at the food regimen. It'll depend upon your scenario or situation.

Work with a dietitian to create an individualized plan. During your low-fiber food regimen, avoid foods that have insoluble fiber and be sure to take note of the fiber content in packaged meals.

Many of the meals allowed on a low-fiber food plan, like pudding and white bread, shouldn't emerge as a staple on your everyday eating regimen, particularly once you begin slowly reintroducing fiber.

Made in United States
Orlando, FL
15 January 2024